Practical Guide to Ear Candling

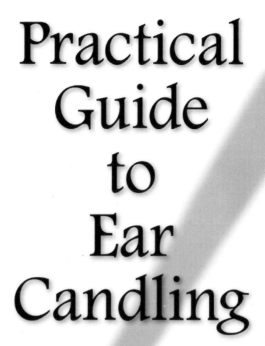

by

Russell Sheppard

D1491266

Evan Feldman & Terry Oquinn
editors

Sixth Edition
2002

Author's Note

Dear Reader,

In publishing this book we have attempted to present the best information possible on the history of the ear candling process and how it may help soothe the ears, the body and the mind. I have tried to describe the natural healing process that takes place in the ear, and how ear candling can provide helpful benefits.

I would like to make one thing perfectly clear. If you experience ear pain, loss of hearing, or any other hearing abnormalities, I highly recommend that you see your doctor or licensed practitioner prior to using ear candles. There are many ear problems that require specific treatment by a doctor. Ear Candling can be a relaxing, soothing, and entertaining experience if and when used correctly in that regard. I do not diagnose or make any medical claims about ear candles. They are not FDA approved, as of yet, nor are they to be used, or considered in any way, as a medical device.

We believe that this booklet will enrich your life and touch the lives of those you love and care for. I hope you enjoy learning and performing the process, and hope you try Wally's ear candling products and will tell others about the benefits you have experienced. Millions of people around the world have used and enjoyed ear candles.

Good luck, good health, and much success in your life!

-Russell Sheppard

P.O. Box 5275
Auburn, CA 95604
www.wallysnatural.com
ISBN 0-9672708-0-4

Contents

Contents

Contents

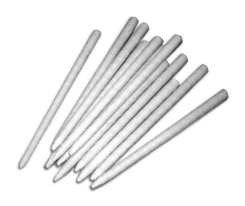

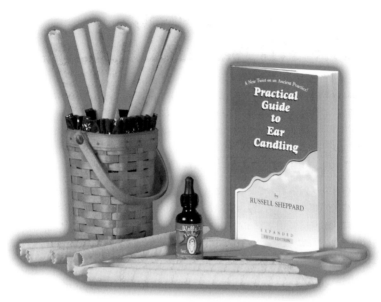

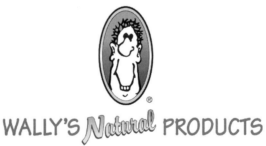

WALLY'S *Natural* PRODUCTS

visit us online at

www.wallysnatural.com

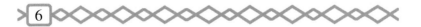

Ear Candling:
The All Natural Process

EAR CANDLING is an age-old "home remedy" used to soothe the ears and to help relieve pain and itching from infections and other conditions. Many people believe the process helps soften earwax and helps the body excrete any excess wax. Other benefits may include helping dry out any fluids in the ear canal.

Ear candling involves the use of a hollow candle coated with wax. The candle is placed gently into the opening of the ear and lit. Warm smoke travels through the candle and soothes the ear. Following the procedure, the ear continues to excrete earwax, plus any extra wax. There should be no discomfort during the procedure or afterward.

Today, ear candling is practiced all over the world. Candle makers now use modern manufacturing techniques, quality control and hygienically sound practices to produce better and more consistent products. As a result, the practice of ear candling is growing even more popular every year!

The process described in this book is soothing, safe and natural if used wisely. If you do not experience the desired effect from ear candling, you may need to consult a physician. Ear candling is a home remedy; it is not a medical procedure. The process may make you feel better and allow your body to heal naturally, but *please use common sense:*

> *Ear candling should <u>not</u> be used as a substitute for medical diagnosis and treatment.*
>
> *If you have a serious ear disease, tubes in your ears, eardrum damage or an upper respiratory infection, consult a physician before you attempt this process.*

Introduction

The Ears May Hold More Mysteries Than We Imagine...

Modern research has determined that many of the supposed "scientific truths" accepted over the past century need to be examined carefully. As we discover more about other cultures and their beliefs, we gain insight into a perspective that has begun to gain acceptance in mainstream scientific investigation.

In medicine, we are learning the value of ancient Chinese herbology and acupuncture. Physicians are experimenting with "positive thinking" to influence the outcome of illnesses for which they have limited treatments available. Many people are consuming organic and natural foods, pure water and supplements that may enhance the immune system and slow the aging process. Spiritual values are having greater influence on many of us.

The future of these trends is unknown, but one conclusion is certain: people will continue to experiment with life-styles and "therapies" that we can't even imagine today. Some will be useless; others may have some effect, though it may be hard to determine.

We suggest that ear candling, with its long history and tradition, has the potential to help and assist people suffering from itching, tinnitus, and impaired hearing. Even more important, the practice can be relaxing and uplifting, leading to a sense of well-being and contentment. In the words of the French physician Alfred A. Tomatis, who dedicated his life to the study of sound and hearing:

> **The ear is a 'royal road' not only for speech but also for all the processes of man's adaptation to self and environment.**
>
> *−The Conscious Ear*

The Origins & Growth of Ear Candling

Spiritual Uses Came First

EAR CANDLING, sometimes known as "ear coning" was used by the Egyptians, Essenes, Chinese, East Indians, and Tibetans over 3,000 years ago. Ancient cultures of North and South America and Lemuria have also been associated with the technique.

Originally the process was described as "coning" because cone-shaped instruments made from pottery clay were used. These glazed pottery cones had a double helix carved inside intended to create a downward spiral flow of smoke from burning herbs into the ear canal.

For centuries, people around the world practiced the art of candling as a form of spiritual healing, to clear the mind and senses. They claimed a person could meditate more deeply and open up their sensitivity. Typically,

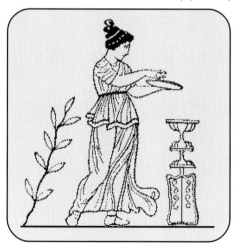

the spiritual leader or shaman of the area would perform a ritual using reeds or clay pottery to heal or improve the person's spiritual condition. In the New World, the Aztec, Mayan, and Native North American cultures all had important rituals involving "ear cones".

The procedure began with those of high social rank, like great warriors, royalty and spiritual leaders, and was used during special initiation rites. Before long, ear candling as a cleansing procedure became common in many early cultures.

History & Background

"Ear Cleansing" Variations

Today ear candles are a popular "home remedy" in Germany, India, Egypt, Mexico, Japan, Australia, Canada, and the United States. People use ear candles to relieve many different types of symptoms of ear problems.

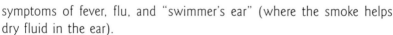

In typical use, the candle is gently placed in the outer ear canal, then the opposite end is ignited to produce smoke and warmth that enters the ear canal, bringing spiritual energy and soothing herbal essences into the ear. This process is also called "Ear Cleansing".

Even people who have never heard of ear candling often blow smoke into the ear canal to relieve symptoms of fever, flu, and "swimmer's ear" (where the smoke helps dry fluid in the ear).

Different materials are used for ear candling around the world. Some Europeans use a pencil-thin cylinder of waxed cloth coated with beeswax.

In South America, both the Spanish and native Indian cultures perform ear coning as a modality for healing the sinuses by "cleansing" the ear canals. They use candles made from rolled-up newspaper that has been waxed and scented with incense one third of the way up from the narrow end of the cone. Mexican Indians also use waxed, rolled-up newspaper with a plug of incense two-thirds down the roll.

Most candles used in North America are made of strips of unbleached 100% cotton or linen soaked in a mixture of hot paraffin, and/or beeswax and herbs or herbal essential oils. The strips are rolled onto a spiral cylinder, excess wax is removed, and then the candles are left to harden.

History & Background

Ear Candling in America

Native American cultures have a long history of using ear candling techniques for spiritual as well as therapeutic effects. Some tribes use hollow twigs or a glazed clay cone, with a double helix carved inside, to create the spiral of smoke. They often use herbs and incense while performing the ritual.

Practitioners of the Choctaw tribe simply blow the smoke of various herbs into the ear canal as a medicinal application, instead of candling the ear or using oils. The Amish culture utilizes a style of ear candling derived from the Cherokee tribe, blowing the smoke of herbs into the ear, rather than burning an ear candle.

There is information available, worldwide, over the internet that promotes ear candling as a method for cleansing the ear canal and sinuses. This information is helpful and beneficial to those people considering ear candling, since in this country ear candling is considered an "alternative" procedure delegated mostly to individuals rather than trained medical practitioners.

Though in the past German medical students have been required to learn ear candling as part of their course of study, in the United States ear candling is practiced without the support of the medical establishment. In fact, physicians and medical organizations have sometimes tried to prevent people from experiencing the process. A few holistic doctors, though, have shifted to using ear candling instead of more invasive irrigation techniques.

> *Though ear candling may not be the answer to all ear, sinus, or throat problems, people have used it to relieve symptoms of itching, congestion and discomfort associated with eye, ear, nose, and throat ailments. With a long tradition around the world, ear candling should continue its popularity to help people in a natural and effective way.*

THE BASICS OF EAR CANDLING

Modern ear candling uses disposable hollow candles made from strips of unbleached cotton or linen dipped in paraffin or beeswax. The spiral roll of these candles creates the same effect as the ancient pottery ear cones. Some candles are made with herbs or essential oils mixed into the wax, in a similar way as the ancients placed herbs in their ear cones for the beneficial effects of the smoke.

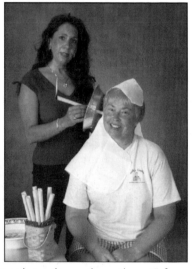

The burning candle creates a gentle, soft flow of warmth and smoke that flows into the ear, drying the ear out, and helping to soften old earwax, and to soothe the ear. The process is very soothing, relaxing and non-invasive. At no point does the tip of the candle or the ear become hot to the touch. In fact, the candle should never burn down closer than 4" from the ear. The procedure is said to assist the body's natural excretion process over a period of time.

Though ear candlers originally thought the candle actually "drew out" earwax through suction, or a vacuum, we now realize that little, if any, of that residue in the candle comes from the ear. Most of the wax found in the candle is probably the result from burning the candle.

If the interior of the burned candle contains a brown powder, however, this could indicate there was not a good seal around the ear. Another candle should be used, making sure it fits properly, and listening for the crackling sound as the candle burns. How you feel, overall, after the ear candling process is also very important.

How Often
Should You Candle?

Ear Candling is used for soothing the symptoms of ear problems and assisting the ear in its natural removal of unwanted, old wax and debris from the ear canal. Because the ear candling process may help the natural elimination of this old earwax, we suggest people allow a day or two between candling sessions.

Use two to four candles per ear during each session. This allows the *slow* candling process to complete a cycle to benefit the ear, which then replenishes its normal protective earwax within a day or so. If you follow this cycle, you can experience candling along with the change of seasons, about four times a year (or as needed).

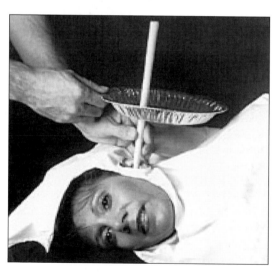

The traditional method of ear candling, in which the person lies on his or her side.

This book describes a new, improved method.

Ear Candling
A New Way!

Ear Candling can aid the normal bodily process of cleansing the ear. For many years, people have promoted ear candling in a horizontal position, lying on one's side, allowing the candle to enter the ear canal in a vertical position.

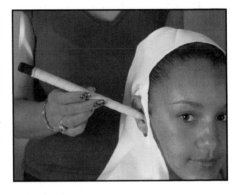

Though this is the traditional method, and we have been pleased with the results, we have conducted research to determine that the effect of **having the person sit up, placing the candle in an angled position about ten degrees tilted above horizontal, is just as effective**.

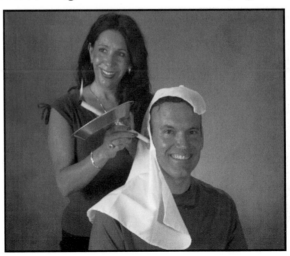

We recommend this position for these reasons:

◆ None of the ash or any other material from the burning candle can fall down into the ear.

◆ The person performing the procedure can direct the smoke more directly into the ear.

◆ The candle can be held directly over a bowl of water to cut off the ash when the candle has burned down to about 4" in length. As the candles burns down, cut the ash off every couple of inches.

◆ Because it takes place sitting up, the process will help drain the sinuses and Eustachian tubes of the person being candled.

◆ As a follow-up to the ear candling session, you may apply a few drops of ear oil to a cotton swab and gently apply the oil to the outside of the ear canal. In this position, the oil will help to soothe the ear.

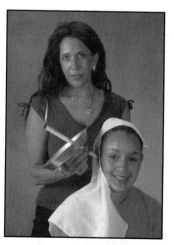

**"Come to the edge," he said.
They said, "We are afraid."
"Come to the edge," he said.
They came.
He pushed them...
And they flew.**

Guillaume Apollinaire

Getting Started

Supplies Needed For Candling

Before you begin, gather the following items:

Wally's *"Edge"* Ear Candles (any variety)	Ear Candles (2-4 per ear)
Scissors	To cut the ash off the candle
Small bowl of water	To extinguish the ash and the candle
Aluminum pie pan	With a hole cut off-center for the candle to fit through
Matches or lighter	To light the candles
Head & shoulder cover, treated with fire retardant (or dampened towels)	To cover the head and upper body and prevent flame from spreading to hair, clothing, bedding or furniture
Wally's Ear Oil	To soothe and protect the ear after candling
Wally's Itch-Away Oil	To relieve itching in the ear after candling
Lotion or massage oil	For the facial massage.
Trash bags	For disposal of the debris

Getting Started

Choosing Ear Candles

Today you can find several types, styles and materials used in ear candles. Made of unbleached cotton (muslin) or linen, ear candles are manufactured by wrapping wax-soaked material onto a cone or cylinder, with a tapered or straight end to fit into the ear. The shape usually resembles a tapered straw or cone.

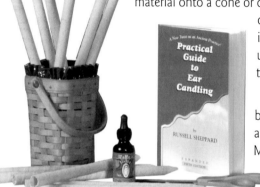

The wax used can be beeswax, paraffin, or a mixture of the two. Many manufacturers also offer candles made with herbs, which can add the benefits of aromatherapy and may help soothe the person being candled.

The color of the candle depends on the fabric and wax used in its manufacture. Variations in the color of wax occur naturally, ranging from pure white to a deep yellow or amber. Some candles contain dyes or natural colorants for a rainbow of different candle colors. You should always try to use ear candles as pure and natural as possible, since some people may react to dyes and allergens contained in certain types of ear candles.

Use extreme caution with ear candles that resemble thin straws or pencils — they could slip too deeply in the ear and push against the eardrum. Be careful if you use ear candles shaped without a tapered tip, since these could allow powder or wax to drip straight into your ear.

The size, thickness and design of the candle will determine how fast and hot the candle will burn. It can take eight to thirty minutes for the average candle to burn. Thickly wrapped candles burn longer.

Candle Varieties

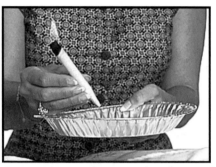

If there is too much wax on the candle it may drip, which could cause problems. Excess wax that might drip inside the candle may cool and block the tapered end near the ear. Some candles come with long skewers that their manufacturer recommends using to clear out the opening — after removing the candle from the ear!

For your safety always leave at least 4" of unburned candle at the bottom, so as not to re-burn any dripped wax inside the candle.

The choice of which type of candle to use is a personal decision, based on an individual's comfort and enjoyment of the process. Some people prefer the all-natural beeswax to a paraffin candle. If you try using different varieties of paraffin and beeswax candles, with or without essential oils added, you can discover the ones that you prefer best.

Ear candles come in many sizes — ranging from a pencil-thin 3/8" diameter candle to a candle greater than 3/4" wide and between 6 and 18 inches in length. The most common candle is a spiral shaped paraffin candle with a tapered end, 1/2" wide by 10" long.

Candle manufacturers usually use natural unbleached fabric, like cotton (muslin) or linen. Fabric comes in different grades, weights and thickness, which will affect the cost and quality of the candles. Muslin cotton may be a coarse weave, making the candles thicker. The fabric could be pre-washed to take out any starch, preventing excess residue or powder from collecting in the candle during its use.

Wally's *"Edge"* Ear Candles are made to burn smoother and longer and are often referred to as "America's Favorite Brand."

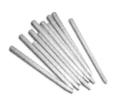

Candle Varieties

The wax used in the candle can be deposited on the outside only, by dipping the candle after it is shaped, or applied both inside and out by dipping the fabric in the wax before it is formed as a candle on a rod. Most of the wax is squeezed off in the manufacturing process, allowing the fabric to become rigid without becoming thick or heavy. As the candle is burned, the amount of wax used in the manufacture should maintain the burning, but not drip out of the candle fabric. Better quality candles burn evenly and slowly, delivering the desired effect through the whole procedure.

Paraffin Candles

The most popular candle sold today is the spiral-wrapped paraffin candle. Paraffin is a man-made wax used in such things as candy bars, and paraffin candles cost less then other candles. This candle works well and is very economical to use. The wax can be on the outside of the candle, or applied both inside and out. Herbs or herbal essential oils can be mixed with the paraffin in the manufacturing process to add a pleasing aroma and other benefits. Sometimes the person being candled may feel a little itching after the process, caused by their reaction to the wax. This feeling should stop after a few hours, or you may use a drop or two of **Wally's Ear Oil** or **Wally's Itch-Away Oil** to soothe the ears.

Beeswax Candles

This candle is better than paraffin for people who have allergies or who desire to use all natural products. The effects are the same as the paraffin candle but should eliminate the chance of an itching reaction after the process. The cost of beeswax is higher, and because beeswax is sticky, it is more difficult to make these candles. They can be made with a spiral or straight wrap, and herbs or herbal essential oils can be mixed with the beeswax for added benefits.

Candle Varieties

Candles Containing Herbal Essential Oils

Herbs and herbal essential oils mixed in the wax (either paraffin or beeswax) during manufacture of a candle will add the herbal benefits to the smoke. These candles can be spiral wrapped, tapered, or straight wrapped (resembling a pencil).

Certain herbal essential oils are useful in relieving some symptoms accompanying colds, flu, and sinus congestion. Other herbs tend to stimulate elimination of mucus, containing residue of the body's attempt to combat infection.

Candles containing herbal essential oils offer pleasant aroma and may be beneficial in soothing and relaxing the person, which may foster the body's natural healing process. Some of the herbs helpful in this regard include lavender, echinacea, eucalyptus, tea tree oil, chamomile, evening primrose, golden seal and sage.

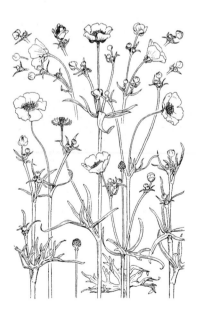 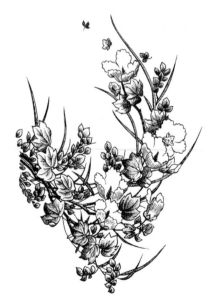

The Ear Candling Process

Two Methods To Consider...

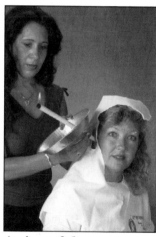

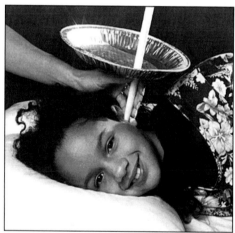

A view of the new, improved method this book describes in detail.

The Tradtional method of ear candling, in which the person lies on his or her side, illustrated above.

WHAT EAR CANDLING CAN DO

◆ This procedure does not necessarily produce healing effects or cure any disease. It may relieve symptoms and can soothe someone's discomfort and it is relaxing.

◆ The process can soften old earwax and may assist the ear in excreting old wax and other material from the ear naturally, for a few days following the procedure. The ear removes wax on it's own, naturally.

◆ The residue left in the candle after its use could be the result of the burning process itself. Burning the ear candle may not "draw out" wax from the ear.

◆ The use of traditional home remedies like ear candling should not substitute for seeking medical attention if symptoms persist or intensify.

◆ Millions of people have reported positive results.

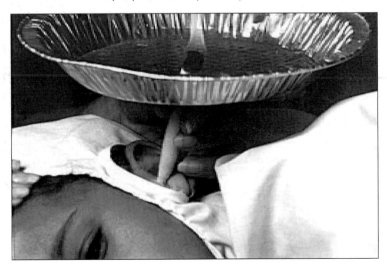

BASIC RULES

◆ *Always use common sense around fire.*

◆ *Do not insert objects or push anything into the ear!*

◆ *Make sure the candle is not jammed into the ear.*

If you follow the traditional method (having the person lie on their side) and anything falls into the ear, stop the procedure and tilt the head to let the material fall out. You can also flush clean water into the ear to rinse out any of this material.

◆ *Do not burn the candle too close to the ear (leave at least 4 inches), and use safe, non-flammable materials (aluminum foil to catch the ash and damp towels over the head and shoulders) to protect from fire.*

◆ *Make sure your area is very clean, and that your supplies are new (or cleaned thoroughly with disinfectant after each use).*

Following this advice will help prevent injury or harm to the ear.

The Process

What to Expect From Ear Candling

During the ear candling process, you may first feel the candle being lightly inserted. Then when it is lit, you may feel a warm sensation in your ear. As the candle burns down you should hear some cracking and popping sounds coming from the candle. This is normal—relax and enjoy the process.

During the ear candling procedure, you might feel a sensation of increased pressure or the sound of your pulse in your ear. This may be the response of nerve endings and sensitive acupuncture points, which connect the ear to other areas of the body. According to the philosophy behind acupuncture, paths called meridians are channels for streams of the *ch'i*, the energy flow that carries our life force. If hearing is impaired, blocked, or pressure placed against the nerves in your ear, you could interrupt that energy flow.

Ear candling also acts to aid your ears by clearing out debris and earwax accumulated over many years. This material may contain evidence of past infections, pollen, ear mites, worms and even parasites.

If you have a hearing loss or a *Candida* infection in your ears, near the end of the procedure you may feel a little heat or a slight discomfort. If this is uncomfortable, you could stop the process and continue another time.

When the candling is completed, you might notice your hearing improves or your head feels lighter, especially if a blockage of wax has moved inside your ear. Your ear(s) could feel airy and more sensitive to subtle sounds and tones. You may experience a sense of wellness, well-being, and "freshness".

Supplies for an
Ear Candling Session

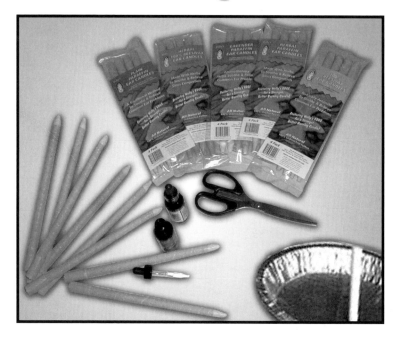

If you feel an itching sensation or slight warmth in your ear(s) after the procedure, you can use a cotton swab (like a Q-tip®) to place a drop or two of **Wally's Ear Oil** or **Wally's Itch-Away Oil** at the entrance to the ear canal, then tipping your head to the side to let the liquid flow into the canal. This can be continued for several days, if necessary.

If you receive a facial massage after the candling, your sinuses may be draining. This can help relieve built-up pressure from materials clogging your sinus passages. The draining usually stops in a couple of days.

A good time to have your ears candled is when the seasons change, or at least twice a year. Use your own judgment to determine how often you wish to have ear candling done.

The Process

THE NEW WAY IS EASY

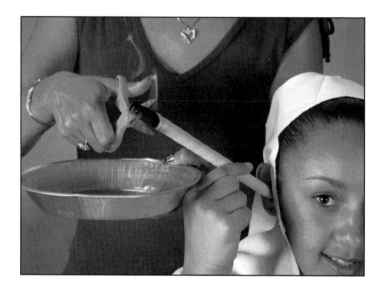

1. Dampen Towels. Place towels over head and around ear.

2. Have person SIT UP.

3. Use aluminum pie pan with hole for candle, angling the candle about 5-10 degrees upward.

4. Light candle, allowing the soothing smoke and warmth from the candle to flow into the ear.

5. Cut candle ash every 2". When the candle burns to about 4" in length, remove from ear and extinguish candle in bowl of water.

6. You may want to use two or more candles for each ear.

7. **Use Wally's Ear Oil to soothe and protect the ears after candling.**

Traditional Method

THE TRADITIONAL PROCEDURE OF EAR CANDLING

The procedure as outlined below has been the usual method of ear candling through hundreds of years. The process is effective, but there is the remote possibility that something could drop into the ear through the candle. *For this reason, Wally's recommends you try the NEW WAY shown earlier in this manual.* This helps to ensure that nothing could drop into the ear.

In either case, we urge you to be very safe around the flame of the candle, and to cover the person's head and upper body with damp towels or flame-resistant covering.

1. **Make sure you have all your supplies before you start the candling process.**

2. **Have the person lie on a massage table, bed, or couch on their side with one ear facing up. Use a pillow to keep the head as level as possible. Some people like a small pillow placed between their knees for their comfort.**

3. **Cover the head and shoulder with moist towels, or any flame-proofed material (such as something treated with fire retardant spray), leaving the ear uncovered.** *Make sure the hair and* 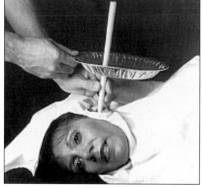 *any facial hair is covered and protected from fire. The person should not have hairspray or other flammable material in their hair.*

Traditional Method

4. Insert the candle through the off-center hole in a pie pan. The hole should be off center to allow for your shoulder. Place the narrow end of the candle 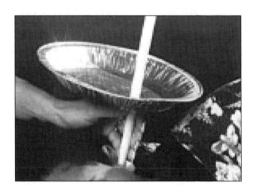 into the ear canal *gently* — it only needs to fit in the opening of the ear to form a seal. Do not press too hard, or you might block the small end of the candle. When you have a comfortable seal, you can light the large end of the candle.

5. *When the candle is lit, make sure there is no smoke escaping from around the bottom of the candle at* 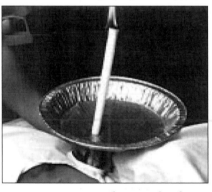 the ear. If this happens, your seal is not secure. Reset the candle by gently pulling the ear around the opening, or rotate the candle very slowly to arrive at a better seal. Do not push the candle any deeper into the opening. If these adjustments do not stop the smoke from escaping, you should remove the candle and start over.

6. *The person should hear crackling sounds during the process.* If not, the tip of the candle may be angled to the side of the ear canal and not down the middle of the ear.

Adjust the angle of the candle as needed. If this doesn't bring back, or start the sound, the bottom of the candle could be clogged with wax. Extinguish the flame, and pull the candle out to check the opening. Always be thoughtful to the comfort of the person being candled.

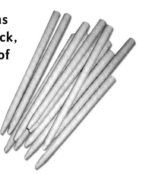

7. When the candle is burning properly, you can begin massaging the face. This can add relief and relaxation for people with sinus problems. Using a small amount of massage oil or lotion, slide your thumb slowly and gently under and over the eye, from the nose to the ear. You can also "walk" two fingers in the same motion. (as shown on page 32, in the diagram *Face Massage*).

8. When the candle has burned down approximately 2" or when the top black ash curls over, put the bowl of water just under the flame. Use scissors to

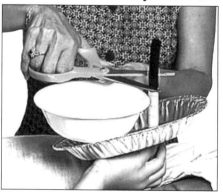

cut the candle from the side just above the flame. Don't push or pull at the candle — just snip it off. The ash should fall to the back into the bowl. *Always be very careful around fire, to make sure no ash or burning embers falls on flammable material!* If the ash does not drop back into the bowl, pick it up with the scissors as quickly as possible. Repeat trimming the ash away while the candle burns, until the candle is about 4" from the bottom.

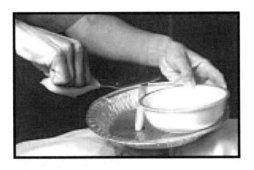

9. When the flame gets down to about four inches from the ear, remove the candle, with the aluminum pan, from the ear, making sure the flame and ash are held over the bowl of water. Pull the candle out of the pan and extinguish it into a bowl of water.

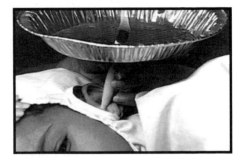

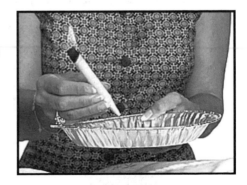

10. *People say that after candling, over the next few days the ear can eject the softened old earwax.* People have also told us they feel better, feel "clean" and "light" inside, and that they may "hear clearer tones" after being candled. This process may not have these or any other effect on all individuals, and Wally's Natural Products makes no claims to any medical benefits from ear candling. Ear candling has been experienced and enjoyed by millions of people around the world.

11. The first candle just gets things going. We recommend you use at least two candles per ear, and up to four per ear. Start the next candle right away for best results. Once finished with the first ear, begin candling the other ear.

12. *Any and all materials that come from ear candling must be disposed of properly, because of possible infections (bacteria, viruses, other microorganisms and their toxins) that may be present. The use of a zip-lock type bag is recommended.*

13. *Be sure to thoroughly wash your hands and wash or disinfect all reusable supplies.*

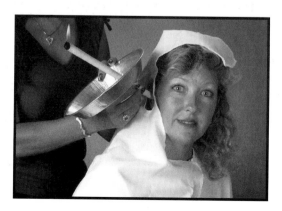

Sinus and Face Massage

The face massage can help open clogged sinuses, feels good, and relaxes the person being candled. This massage can also help stimulate the sinuses for draining material collected within these cavities. Some of that material may include products of infection and other fluid buildup. People with sinus problems can have the massage done at anytime.

Just before starting the candling, rub the outer ear and scalp gently for about 30 seconds to open up circulation in the ear and facial areas.

There are two ways to massage the face. One is to rub the area gently using the thumb. The other uses the index and middle finger in a "walking" motion, keeping a constant pressure as you move (in the direction of the arrows on the diagram) from the nose to the ear. Follow the sequence described on this page.

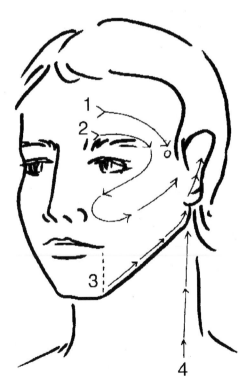

Keep the comfort and pleasure of the person in mind while doing the face massage, and make sure your finger nails are short to prevent scratching or discomfort.

During Candling

1. Start above the nose, working across the upper eye and down to the temple.

2. Beginning at the top of the eyebrow, work your way to the cheek bone and around the bottom of the eye, then go down under the cheek to the ear.

3. Starting at the chin now work your way up the jaw bone to the ear.

4. Start at the lower neck and go up the neck to the back of the ear.

After the ear candling session, you may also massage the scalp (without lotion or oil, if the person prefers) to relax the individual.

Sinusitis

The single most important step in bringing relief is to clear the sinuses and nasal passages of mucus and any germs the mucus has trapped. Three symptoms common to sinusitis cases are a clogged nose, a continuing flow of mucus down the throat, and often a headache.

It is often beneficial to use a soothing lotion on the face during this massage. You might try a light, aromatic, non-greasy massage oil or lotion.

> Take what you can use
> And let the rest go by.
>
> *Ken Kesey*

Anecdotes

What Some People Have Told Us

No claims are made for these accounts. They are presented here as examples of experiences people have shared with us over the years.

Dozens of people have reported no longer needing hearing aids, or having to turn them down, after several sessions of candling. Many have been helped with sinus and allergy symptoms after the facial massage and the ear candling session. After several candling sessions, quite a few people have reported that the ringing, buzzing and/or itching of their ears stopped or was less than they had suffered before.

One man had terrible headaches along with tension in his neck and shoulders. After several ear candling sessions he stopped taking all his pain medications, because his headaches were gone.

A 36-year old woman, a secretary in a large office, found it more and more difficult to use the telephone with her right ear. Her problem had been building up over a three-year period. She had a feeling of "blockage" and sounds appeared to be muffled. Otoscopic examination revealed the right external auditory canal to be completely blocked with earwax. After the ear was candled, her "blocked" feeling disappeared after a few days.

A man came back for another session of candling, and while on the bed he started to cry. He told me that after 10 years of not being able to hear, one session opened up his ear. For the first time he could hear the water running down the drain in the shower. He could also hear the keys in his pocket, and he also told us he had to turn down his hearing aids.

Again, we make no claims or guarantee the results, if any at all, anyone will or will not receive with ear candling, but we continue to be amazed at the positive results reported from the millions of people who have used them.

THE EAR

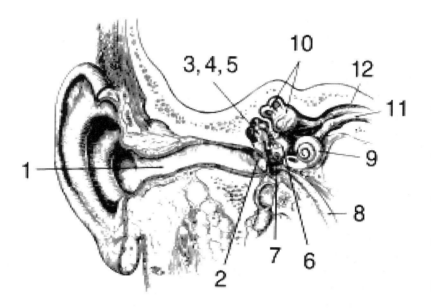

1. External canal	6. Oval window
2. Eardrum	7. Round window
(tympanic membrane)	8. Eustachian tube
The Ossicle:	9. Cochlea
3. Malleus	10. Semicircular canal
4. Incus	11. Auditory nerve
5. Stapes	12. Vestibular nerve

The Ear

Anatomy of the Ear

The ear consists of three main sections: the external ear, the middle ear and the inner ear. Each performs a specific function in receiving, amplifying and transmitting hundreds of thousands of tones rapidly and efficiently to the brain, which interprets these as sound.

Disorders of the outer ear are not usually serious. The middle ear, though, can get bacterial and viral infections (*otitis media*). Disorders of the very delicate organs of the inner ear (the *cochlea* and *labyrinth*) can be much more serious, since the inner ear also plays a special role in the maintenance of our balance.

The Outer Ear

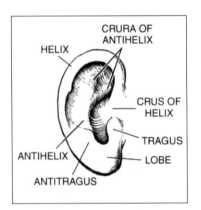

The outer ear includes the parts of the ear we see—folds of skin and cartilage known as the *pinna* or *auricle*. This structure captures sound and directs it into the ear canal, a passage about 3/4 inch long that leads from the *pinna* to the eardrum.

The ear canal funnels sound waves toward the eardrum. The skin lining it contains glands which produce *cerumen* (earwax), a waxy substance that protects the ear canal and ear drum. The body replenishes new ear wax approximately every 24 hours. Little hairs, called *cilia*, line the ear canal and direct the flow of *cerumen* away from the eardrum, carrying other material that sticks to it. This mixture may contain remains of infection, dead cells, pus, blood, pollen and other plant matter, dust and dirt, bacteria, viruses, mold and fungi. As *cerumen* flows naturally out of the ear canal, the ear is protected from the adverse effects of these waste materials and contaminants.

The Ear

If the canal becomes infected, it can produce pain and discharge or become blocked with excess wax, causing discomfort or pain along with hearing problems. This may lead to serious health problems and require medical attention.

The Middle Ear

The cavities of the middle and inner ear are both contained in the *temporal bone*, which forms a part of the side wall and base of the skull. The main organs of the middle ear are the eardrum, or *tympanic membrane*, which is a broad, flat, cone-shaped membrane about 1/2 inch in diameter and less than 1/50th of an inch thick. This membrane covers the entrance to the middle ear cavity and connects to the three tiniest bones in the body (known as the hammer, anvil and the stirrup), collectively called the *ossicle*.

These bones form a bridge that connects the eardrum with the oval window, an opening in the wall of the middle ear that leads to the inner ear. The interconnected *ossicle* triples the incoming sound pressure and converts airborne sound energy from the outer ear to mechanical energy in the middle ear. The sound energy pressure is amplified 30 times as it becomes concentrated on the oval window.

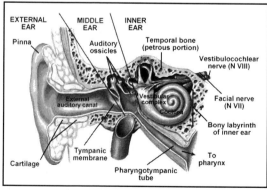

The middle ear is connected to the back of the throat (*pharynx*) by the *Eustachian tube*, which permits the passage of air (as well as bacteria, viruses and parasites) from the nose. The *Eustachian tube* is vital in keeping the middle ear air pressure equal to the outside air, but is also a common source of spreading infections to the ear.

The Ear

The Inner Ear

The inner ear opens from the middle ear via the oval window. It is a snail-shaped chamber lined with tiny hairs and filled with fluid of the *vestibule*.

The lower part of the inner ear is the spiral-shaped *cochlea* (the Latin word for "snail shell" which it resembles) and is about the size of a finger tip. Movements of this fluid in response to vibrations from the *ossicle* are transmitted through the *auditory* (or eighth) nerve, which leads to the brain, where the hearing process is completed. Damage to the *cochlea* can result in *Tinnitus* (noises in the ear) or deafness.

The *labyrinth* is a group of fluid-filled *semicircular canals*, three connected tubes bent into half circles, connected to the *vestibular* nerve that leads to the brain. This structure, in the center and upper part of the inner ear, is essential to balance. Disorders of the *labyrinth* include viral infection (*Labyrinthitis*) as well as *Meniere's disease*, an increase in the amount of fluid in the canals. Both may produce dizziness, nausea, loss of hearing and loss of balance or vertigo.

There is more information regarding both *Tinnitus* and *Labyrinthitis* at the end of this chapter.

Functions of the Ear

The primary functions of the ear are hearing and balance. A diagram on the next page illustrates how the hearing process works.

In the inner ear, the semicircular canals function to maintain balance. Tiny hairs, called *cilia*, line these structures and send the sensations of movement and head position to the brain through the *vestibular nerve*. Infections, fluid build-up and other conditions present in the middle ear will sometimes affect this vital function of the inner ear, which can produce problems with the sense of balance.

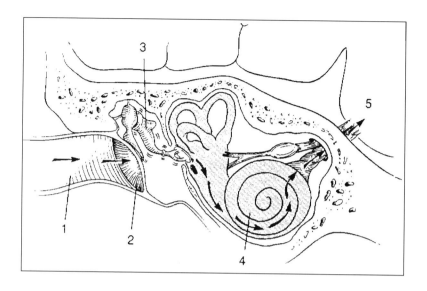

How You Hear

Sound waves are captured by the auricle and enter the ear canal (1) where they strike the eardrum (2) and make it vibrate.

These vibrations are transmitted through the ossicular chain (3), three small bones (malleus, incus and stapes) in the middle ear.

The stapes is connected to the oval window on the cochlea (4), a coiled labyrinth in the inner ear filled with liquid and lined with microscopic hairs (cilia) in a structure called the organ of corti.

Sensory impulses stimulated by nerve endings in the cochlea pass to the brain via the auditory nerve (5).

Ear Ailments

Middle Ear Infections
(Otitis Media)

The middle ear is a small space between the outer and the inner ear. Air pressure is kept constant by the *Eustachian tube*, which enters the middle ear from the back of the nasal cavity. When bacteria or viruses invade the middle ear, infections commonly result in soreness or pain, inflammation, and a buildup of fluids.

The *ossicular chain* must be surrounded by air to function properly. If fluid fills the middle ear, the effectiveness of these bones can be greatly reduced because their movements in transmitting and amplifying sound energy is impaired by the resistance of fluids.

Children are particularly prone to this because their *Eustachian tubes* are short and follow a more horizontal direction. Thus, infections in children (*otitis media*) can easily reach the middle ear from the nasal cavity. Children may also have fluids accumulate due to the presence of large amounts of adenoidal tissue.

Otitis media remains a major public health problem in the world today, with costs for treatment estimated at more than $2 billion annually. It is the most common medical problem for children. More than 19 million persons are afflicted with hearing disabilities, including over 4 million school age children.

One of the foremost experts in the study of *otitis media* in the United States is Jack L. Paradise, M.D. Professor of Pediatrics and Community Medicine, University of Pittsburgh School of Medicine, and Medical Director of the Ambulatory Care Center, Children's Hospital of Pittsburgh. Paradise says:

> "Perhaps we have reduced the number of serious illnesses that come from *otitis media*, but only at the price of increasing the number of patients with chronic disease, which has in turn led to an ever increasing number of surgical procedures to treat and prevent *otitis media*."

Ear Ailments

What does this mean in terms of numbers?

◆ **Thirty million visits per year to doctors are estimated to take place for the treatment of otitis media at an estimated cost of $120 for each episode.**

◆ **One study estimated that on any given day in the U.S. up to 30 percent of all children are suffering an ear infection or an abnormal middle ear condition. That means that up to 900,000 children a day are suffering an ear-related condition.**

◆ **Before age six, 90 percent of all children in the U.S. will have had at least one ear infection. Half of the children who have had one ear infection before the age of one will have six or more episodes before the age of three.**

The Causes of Middle Ear Infections

The single most frequent factor causing ear infections is poor *Eustachian tube* function resulting in inadequate ventilation of the middle ear. The cause depends on the type of infection or *otitis media*.

Secretory otitis media occurs when fluids resulting from colds or allergies enter the middle ear by way of the *Eustachian tube*. *Acute serous otitis media* is caused by a bacterial or viral infection leading to the accumulation of fluids. *Acute purulent otitis media* may follow if pus from the bacterial infection builds up, which could lead to a ruptured eardrum. *Chronic otitis media* is caused by the lingering presence of an untreated bacterial infection, infected adenoids, or problems with the *Eustachian tube*.

Middle ear infections are not dangerous when treated promptly. Temporary hearing loss can occur during the infection, but hearing should return as the fluids drain. Ear infections tend to recur, especially if there are infected adenoids. An untreated infection could lead to a ruptured eardrum, pain and loss of hearing.

Ear Ailments

Symptoms of Middle Ear Infections:

◆ Temporary hearing loss, sometimes accompanied by a stuffy or clogged feeling in the ear.

◆ Fever, glassy eyes, loss of appetite and general fussiness, especially if the person has a cold.

◆ Acute, stabbing pain in the ear. Babies often will rub or tug at the ear while prolonged crying takes place.

◆ Nausea and/or vomiting.

◆ Bleeding or discharge of pus from the ear. These symptoms could mean the eardrum has ruptured to relieve the pressure from fluid build-up.

A Word About Children

Parents can prevent some of their children's ear infections by teaching them to *wipe (instead of blowing)* their noses when they have a cold. A child's ear infection can become very painful, and should be treated very early. Medical care usually includes antibiotics and sometimes careful draining of the fluids built up in the ear. Some of the procedures used by physicians may be painful and traumatic to a child.

Do not candle the ears of children experiencing high fever, vomiting or diarrhea associated with serious illness.

EARACHE

The term earache is often used when describing the pain that accompanies an ear infection. An earache can be caused when infected fluid accumulates in the middle ear and exerts pressure against the eardrum. As the fluid increases in volume, it pushes more and more against the pliable eardrum, stretching it to its breaking point. It will also occur when the *tympanic membrane* has ruptured, spilling contaminated material into the ear canal.

Pain felt in the ear does not necessarily originate in the ear itself. Because there are many delicate nerve connections between the ear and the nose, mouth and throat, earaches may be caused by a variety of conditions, including changes in air pressure, *tonsillitis*, dental problems and infected sinuses and adenoids.

Middle ear infections (*acute otitis media*) are associated with upper respiratory infections (colds, flu, allergies) and draining sinuses that travel through the *Eustachian tube* from the *nasopharynx*, which is the space directly behind the nose.

The *Eustachian tube* is a narrow canal about the diameter of a pencil with collapsible walls. This tube opens hundreds of times a day, allowing air to enter the canal and travel to the middle ear, usually with every third swallow and with every yawn. If the tube becomes blocked, fluids and pus produced by an infection cannot drain from the ear, causing hearing loss by inhibiting the vibration of the eardrum.

Improper nose-blowing, or sniffing germ-laden mucus from the nose back into the throat can cause inflammation or blockage of the *Eustachian tube*. Middle ear infections are caused directly by bacteria or viruses, or indirectly by the presence of pneumonia, influenza (cold), measles, scarlet fever or mumps in the upper respiratory area.

Ear Ailments

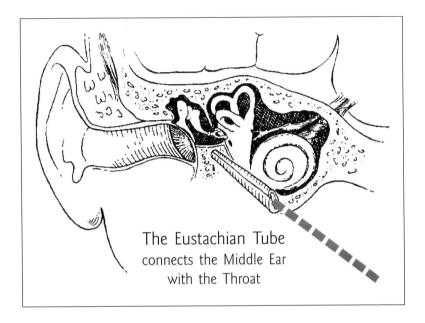

The Eustachian Tube
connects the Middle Ear
with the Throat

The three main functions of the *Eustachian tube* are:

1. To ventilate the middle ear

2. To allow fluid to drain into the throat

3. To protect the middle ear from anything blown from the throat

Malfunctions are:

1. "Floppy"– when the tube does not close properly

2. The tube becomes obstructed or swollen

3. The tube's angle doesn't allow fluid to drain

Ear Ailments

Treatments for Earwax Problems

Many procedures used to treat *ceruminosis* — the term used for earwax accumulation, impaction, and infection — have not been very effective, and in fact, some can cause damage to the ear. Some prescription drugs, particularly those containing hydrogen peroxide, have been known to irritate the skin of the ear canal. Water, used by doctors and home ear flushing kits, can cause earwax to swell rapidly and injure the eardrum, the ear canal, or the sensitive structure of the middle ear.

Beware the Cotton-Tipped Swab!

One of the most dangerous earwax removal methods involves the use of cotton-tipped swabs which people often poke and jab into their ears. The most common object causing damage to the *tympanic membrane* and *ossicular chain* was a cotton-tipped applicator.

In addition to hearing loss, people can suffer symptoms like dizziness, bleeding, vomiting, and often severe pain. Not only is the risk of permanent ear damage high in using the swabs, but the swabs are not effective. Earwax that can be dislocated by them is usually on its way to falling out of the ear of its own accord. The harder sticky earwax is only compacted more deeply in the ear by pressing the swab against it.

> *Swabs are meant to be used on the outside of the ear only.*
> *Read the package and follow the instructions.*
> *Never put a hard object into the ear!*

Ear Ailments

Impacted Earwax & Its Removal

Treatment Alternatives

Earwax accumulation is a common cause of deafness among American adults, though it is often overlooked by doctors, according to a recent article in the *Journal of Occupational Medicine* by Dr. James Kawchak. Children with ear problems are often seen by physicians, though typical medical procedures (ear tubes, irrigation with warm water, or other invasive techniques) may be painful and traumatic to a child.

The increased pollution of our environment has had a very pronounced effect on hearing difficulties. Normally, the ear eliminates earwax spontaneously, but dust and dirt particles in the air can adhere to the sticky wax, creating a substance not easily expelled naturally. Instead of acting as a defense against infection, earwax may become an infecting and troublesome substance itself.

A sensation of blockage in the ear may be associated with earwax or fluids. Natural secretions from the *ceruminous glands* in the outer ear may accumulate and harden to form earwax.

In most cases, *cerumen* impaction is self-induced through ill-advised attempts at cleaning the ear. If you pull on your earlobe and the pain worsens, this could be caused by an infection in the outer ear canal.

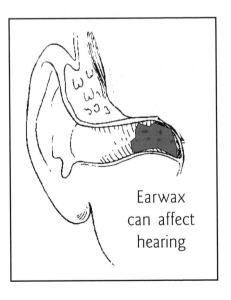

Earwax can affect hearing

Ear Ailments

You should never use cotton swabs or your finger to remove the wax. Ear candling works to warm the area, allowing the earwax to soften. This helps the ear excrete the old, hard accumulation of earwax naturally, over the next day or two, usually while at sleep, without using invasive or painful procedures.

If the condition requires it, impacted earwax can be removed by a doctor using various tools, such as scraping, vacuuming, surgery and flushing. The most common method of removing earwax is to use an ear syringe with warm water.

To avoid pushing the wax up against your eardrum, the doctor directs the stream of a warm solution into the roof of each ear canal. This can cause some discomfort and pain, and the procedure can also damage the eardrum itself. The eardrum is a very delicate part of the body and is not intended to withstand such a direct force.

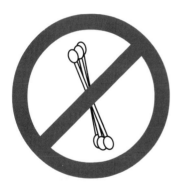 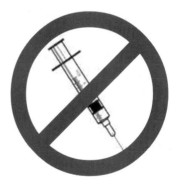

Never try to clean or remove an object from the ear with a cotton swab, bobby pin, key or any other hard object. These can cause damage to the outer ear, or even perforate your eardrum. A sharp object could even damage the tiny bones (*ossicular chain*) in the middle ear, which could lead to hearing impairment.

Foreign bodies (including insects, airborne seeds, or small objects) may find their way into the ear. The use of ear candles may also be helpful in relieving pain and soreness from these problems, allowing the ear to cleanse itself of these irritants.

Ear Ailments

Tinnitus

Describing the misery of *tinnitus* is not easy. This condition is the perception of abnormal ear or head noises. There is actually a physical basis for most *tinnitus*. In nature, absolute silence does not exist. Normally, when external sound is absent, your ears may detect sounds of your body processes (heartbeat, breathing, digestion, etc.) A constant wide range of sound levels in the ear, like ringing, buzzing, hissing are called *tinnitus*.

Your hearing can suffer from this interference. These sounds may be the result of damage to the *cochlea*, the most sensitive component of the hearing mechanism. Most of the time this is a permanent discomfort caused by nerve damage. Severe headaches and stress can be contributory also.

"*Exotic tinnitus*" comes from disorders of organs near the auditory apparatus. One possible cause of these noises is the contraction of an ear muscle or movement of the soft palate, the tongue or the uvula at the back of the throat. Vascular noises (of the circulatory system) are the most common cause of all, though they may result from some physical incapacity. In the case of "*entotic tinnitus*" the noises are often accompanied by deafness to external sounds.

Sometimes the accumulation of wax, fluids, or foreign objects in the ear can lead to dizziness and *tinnitus*. Where inflammation or infections occur in the middle and inner ear, *tinnitus* may be present. Ear candling may relieve some of the pain and other discomfort associated with *tinnitus* and may speed up the natural healing process of the ear. As youth, take care of your ears by avoiding very loud music at concerts, and heavy machinery noises. What we do as a youth, to our bodies, will determine the quality of life as we get older.

Wear earplugs that will help insulate the ear from these noises.

Ear Ailments

Labyrinthitis

The inner ear's *semicircular canals* can become infected by bacteria or viruses and disturb your sense of balance. This condition, known as *labyrinthitis*, causes feelings of nausea and extreme vertigo (a spinning, dizzy sensation). It is either a sensation of motion when there is no motion, or an exaggerated sense of motion in response to a given bodily movement.

When the disease is bacterial, there can be a total loss of hearing on the affected side. The viral form is usually self-limiting and often inappropriately diagnosed for any disease characterized by dizziness. In the vast majority of patients with *labyrinthitis Syndrome*, the acute episode is self-limiting and usually lasts anywhere from days to weeks. Spontaneous recovery is the rule. However, recurrences are common, especially in the first five years following the first episode. In rare cases the episode can last months or even years.

Meniere's disease

Meniere's disease is an affliction of the inner ear, which includes the following symptoms:

- **Loss of hearing**
- **Ringing of the ears**
- **Dizziness and nausea**
- **Distortion of sound**
- **Feeling of pressure in the inner ear**

In this condition there may be an increase of pressure or imbalance of fluid in the inner ear. This syndrome can also be from hemorrhage of the small, delicate parts of the *semicircular canals*. These symptoms can put pressure on the membrane of the *labyrinth* wall, affecting both balance and hearing.

Conclusion

At the library you can find many books on the ear and your body. Here are a few to look for:

Ear Infections In Your Child

Complete Home Medical Guide

The American Medical Association Family Medical Guide

Medical Diagnosis and Treatment

The Encyclopedia of Common Diseases

The Time-Life Medical Advisor

EAR CANDLING: A TRADITIONAL "HOME REMEDY"

Common symptoms or problems affecting the ears are ear infections, earaches, hearing difficulties, *Tinnitus* (constant sounds in the ear) and *Labyrinthitis* (a spinning sensation). Some ear problems affect only the structural parts of the ear, while other symptoms affect hearing as well.

Although ear problems can be distressing and can affect how we perceive the world around us, most are not a serious cause for concern. In many cases, someone could receive positive benefits and could get some relief from pain and discomfort by using the ear candling process. No claim is made for any cure of any disease or ailment, nor that ear candling will relieve any symptoms. How the user views and uses the information in this book is solely up to them.

Good Luck, Have Fun and Enjoy the Process!

Questions & Answers

Common Questions About Ear Candling

1) What is earwax?

Earwax, medically is known as *cerumen*, is a natural substance excreted by glands in the ear canal, which provides a chemical barrier to infection and a physical barrier preventing material from entering the ear. The ear is constantly replenishing *cerumen* for protection against the elements.

Earwax can build up, eventually affecting hearing by muffling sounds from reaching the eardrum. Use of a cotton swab or other hard object in the ear may only push the wax farther into the ear canal, causing more severe problems and could lead to deafness.

2) How can I tell the difference between earwax and drainage of the middle ear?

Earwax is oily and tan to brown in color. Drainage from the middle ear is sticky, yellowish or green in color, and may have a foul odor. When ear candling, there may be candle wax accumulation in the bottom of the candle, which may range from off-white to gray-brown in color.

3) What symptoms come from excess earwax?

Deafness, *tinnitus*, dizziness, echo sensation, headaches and severe earaches are only a few symptoms of *ceruminosis*. The earwax may trap fluids and cause pressure on the eardrum, even leading to damage to this vital organ. If earwax gets lodged beyond the isthmus of the ear, it could cause a reflex cough.

Disturbance in the behavioral patterns in people has been linked to excess *cerumen* (earwax) accumulation in both ears. In some cases, the earwax was impacted to an extent that general anesthesia was necessary to remove it. "If you can eliminate even a little of the old, hard cerumen, you can experience great changes in behavior."

This poses and interesting question: *How many children who are having problems in school or older people who are thought to be "senile" instead may have a hearing problem, perhaps impacted earwax?*

4) Does it take more then one person to ear candle?

Yes! In the traditional method, a person being candled lies on his or her side with their head on a pillow. Another person must watch over the process and cut the ash from the burning candle as needed.

The new method recommended in this booklet has the person sit up, allowing the candle to be placed in an angled position, almost horizontal, where the Candler can easily monitor the progress and avoid problems with ash or fire.

Never do ear candling by yourself.

5) Who can benefit most from ear candling?

We all can! Ear candling can soothe and relieve anyone (including pets) who suffers from ear infections, ear pain, itchy ears, ringing of the ears, hearing loss, *Candida*, yeast or fungus infections.

Common earwax buildup can muffle hearing for many people. Ear candling can help the body eliminate this buildup naturally. This helps the body combat any infections, can restore hearing, and may relieve tension or pressure in the ear from the built-up or impacted *cerumen*.

Candida can cause an allergic reaction, which may lead to itching inside the ear. Parasites can also cause many problems if allowed to grow. "Swimmer's ear" is quite often caused by water being trapped in the ear by earwax, which could host a variety of bacterial or fungal infections and complications.

Questions & Answers

6) Is ear candling uncomfortable?

Ear candling is a soothing, relaxing process, especially using the new technique in which the person sits up while undergoing the ear candle procedure. The only unusual part of the process is the crackling sound as the candle burns down. Some people are amused by all the commotion the process seems to generate. Have fun and enjoy the process!

People that have had damage to the eardrum or have a bad case of *Candida* infection may, in some cases, feel a small amount of discomfort for a very short time. If so, you may want to stop, or try again later.

7) How and where can I learn to do ear candling?

You can learn about ear candling by reading this booklet and by following the instructions carefully. You can also try to find a qualified ear candler in your area and see if they teach the process.

8) How long does it take to learn how to candle?

Whether you learn from this book or a short instruction sheet, you will need to understand the material and feel comfortable with the process before you try it. You also need to gather all the supplies for the ear candling. If you take a training course from a ear candler, make sure you ask about their experience and get references.

Most people learn the technique in two or three sessions, but experience with many people and in different situations is the best teacher. The different responses you will receive from a variety of people can help you understand the process better. Experience is always the best teacher.

9) Why have I not heard or read more about ear candling?

Because the medical establishment in the U.S. has not supported ear candling ans other homeopathic teachings, or research into whether

Questions & Answers

they are effective, people have had to practice the technique quietly, without advertising or promoting the procedure. Only recently, since the internet has become so popular a form of communicating between people, have ear candlers and suppliers been able to get their message out.

Unfortunately there is a lot of quackery and excessive claims on some of the internet sites, but Wally's has always been dedicated to providing accurate information as well as wholesome, safe and natural products for the enjoyment and health of our customers.

A lot of doctors do not want people to use home remedies. Most ear doctors haven't even heard of ear candling. If they have heard of ear candling they don't fully understand the process and are not willing to try it. Instead they will flush, scrape, vacuum, insert tubes and prescribe medication for you at an inflated cost.

Ear candling is considered a "home remedy" that has helped millions of people for hundreds of years, all over the world.

10) How long does an ear candling session take?

When an experienced ear candler does the process, the session usually lasts an hour or more. Each candle takes approximately 8-12 minutes to burn down no closer than 4" from the ear.

You can do one to three sessions over a week's time to get the results you want, but remember to *wait at least 24 hours between sessions, allowing the ear to replace fresh cerumen and not overwhelm the ear.*

11) How many ear candles can be used per session?

If your family doctor or licensed medical practitioner recommends candling a young child or infant, make sure to use *no more than 1/2 to 1 candle per ear.* If more candling is needed, wait at least 24 hours between sessions.

For a young adult to an adult, 2 to 4 ear candles per ear are recommended per session. Never exceed 4 candles per ear in any one candling session, as the ear canal may get irritated and become red and swollen. You may use more candles within 24 hours to get the desired results.

12) How often can a person be candled?

A person with a problem can have candling done in two sessions, 24 hours apart. It takes the ear about 24 hours to replace its protective coating of earwax. Therefore it is not advisable to be candled every day or to use too many candles in one day. Use **Wally's Ear Oil** after being candled to help soothe the ear and protect it from cold and the elements.

The procedure can be done as often as the change of seasons, or as far apart as once or twice a year. Each person has to decide how frequently they feel candling is needed. Men seem to have a lot more earwax and can be candled about every 3 to 4 months. You should always use common sense and your own experience as the determining factor.

13) What should one do right after ear candling?

The first thing to do is put one drop of **Wally's Ear Oil** into the ear to soothe the ear and protect the tender ear canal from cold air and the elements. This helps prevent ear infections. If the ear becomes itchy you can use a drop or two of **Wally's Itch-Away Oil** for natural relief.

Immediately after the ear candling procedure, you should refrain from immersing your head and ears in water for up to 24 hours. You may feel like staying calm and taking it easy while your ears respond to the process.

14) At what age can ear candling be administered?

Though candling has been performed on small babies, we do not recommend this process for children or small infants unless it is approved and suggested by your family physician, pediatrician, licensed medical professional, homeopathic or naturopathic therapist.

Questions & Answers

Ear candling has been very successful in the elderly. A woman 98 years old could no longer hear. She had her ears candled and found that heavy wax buildup was the cause of blockage that made her hard of hearing. This is a common condition among the elderly, and ear candling may be helpful in relieving discomfort, stuffiness and other feelings due to years of neglecting routine ear care. Hearing aids may also cause the ears to build up more wax.

15) Are there people who should not be candled?

People who have had recent ear or sinus surgery as well as bleeding, tubes, or draining of fluids from the ear should not have ear candling done. Any current serious ear or sinus problem should always be referred to a doctor.

If you are not sure or if you have unanswered questions, we recommend that you not have the candling process done. Consult a homepathic or naturopathic therapist.

16) Are there spiritual benefits from being candled?

There is a considerable amount of writing and personal belief on the spiritual aspects of ear candling. People have described an amazing clarity and calmness that came over them after being candled. Some have even said they felt a better sense of overall balance in their life.

In early days of candling this balance is what they first sought, sort of a cleansing of the soul. These claims cannot be proven, but a person should evaluate his or her feelings with regard to their own beliefs.

17) Where can I purchase ear candles and supplies?

Wally's Ear Candles and accessories as well as other ear candle varieties are available at many natural foods stores, through magazines or on the internet. For ordering from internet sources and learning about new products and specials, visit our website at   www.wallysnatural.com or go to your server and type in "ear candles".

Questions & Answers

18) Is there a Certificate or License for ear candling?

Currently, the FDA does not regulate home remedies, and there is no license required. You should, however, follow local regulations and have abusiness license if appropriate. If you take a course in ear candling from an experienced candler, you may receive a certificate of training. If you are interested in starting an ear candling business, this manual will help you learn more about the ears and the ear candling.

19) What is that stuff in the bottom of the candle ?

Most of what you see remaining in the bottom of the ear candle after its use comes from the process of burning the candle. For many years people claimed that ear candles extracted earwax by suction from burning the candle, but that is usually not the case.

I believe if you don't have a very good seal at the ear you will get a lot of powder. Ear candling aids the ear in its natural wax removal, so that for a day or two after being candled your body will remove old, excess earwax that the candling helped soften.

The relaxed and comforting feeling that you feel during and after the ear candling process is part of the entire experience.

Wally's Natural Products

> The great thing in this world
> is not so much where we are,
> but in what direction
> we are moving.
>
> Oliver Wendell Holmes

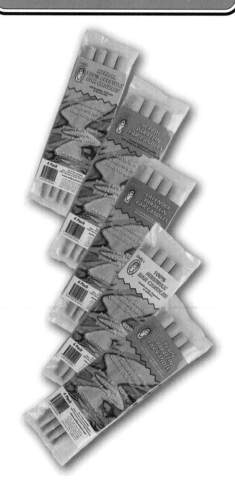

About Wally's Products

Wally's Natural Products has gone to great lengths to provide you with the best quality personal care products, which are available in natural foods stores, natural pharmacies, and mail-order catalogs. If you have access to the internet, check out our website at **www.wallysnatural.com** to learn more about our products and where to find them.

Our five kinds of ear candles are packaged in 2-packs, 4-packs, 12-packs and in bulk. These include the popular Lavender Paraffin, Plain Paraffin and Herbal Paraffin kinds, as well as our wonderful 100% Beeswax and Herbal 100% Beeswax varieties. All varieties feature Wally's new "Edge" construction, making the candle stronger and longer burning. The spiral shape of Wally's Candles causes the smoke to be pulled down into the ear canal. The tapered, individually hand-finished "comfort tip", makes Wally's ear candles comfortable to use and provides reliable, consistent performance.

We suggest you compare the results of paraffin versus beeswax, and to experience the aromatic, soothing herbal blends with their benefits. Wally's paraffin is the finest food-grade variety, and our beeswax is closely monitored and inspected for quality and consistency.

We also furnish accessories like this guide, and our Ear Oil and Itch-Away Oil to compliment your ear candling experience.

Working with herbalists and aromatherapy specialists we have developed a revolutionary line of herbal essential oil blends. Wally's Ear Oil is useful both before and after ear candling, and has been effective soothing earaches and ear discomfort at other times.

Wally's Itch-Away Oil has a unique herbal infusion carried in an oil blend, which has been designed to treat itching in the ears as well as all over the body. This product helps relieve itching from sunburn, poison oak, poison ivy and other plants, insect bites, skin irritations and rashes, and even hemorrhoidal itching. We offer it in a one-ounce dropper bottle (soon available in a spray). It is perfect for camping or other outdoor uses.

Wally's Natural Products

Notes

Dates I Have Ear Candled

Month/Day/Year	Month/Day/Year	Month/Day/Year

Index

Index

Index

Index